Raise kids with ASD:

All You Need to Know About Parenting a Child with ASD.

Katherina C. Norton

Table of Contents

Chapter 1

Understand ASD

Autism spectrum disorder: what is it?
A range of neurodevelopmental diseases known as an autism spectrum disorder (ASD) has an impact on how individuals behave, learn, and interact with others in social situations. People may exhibit recurring, distinctive behavioral patterns or specific interests. These symptoms, which are often present from early infancy and have an impact on everyday functioning, may not be present in all individuals with ASD. ASD may affect both children and adults.

The word "spectrum" describes the vast variety of symptoms, abilities, and degrees of functional dysfunction that may exist in individuals with ASD. While some children and people with ASD are entirely capable of carrying out all everyday activities, others need significant assistance to do even the most basic tasks. Extreme intellectual prowess and severe assistance are both possible in learning and thinking. Asperger syndrome, childhood disintegrative disorder, and pervasive developmental disorders not otherwise specified (PDD-NOS) are all classified as parts of autism spectrum disorder (ASD) in the Diagnostic and Statistical Manual of Mental Disorders (DSM-5, released in 2013). An evaluation of intellectual disability and linguistic impairment is part of an ASD diagnosis.

Every racial and ethnic group, as well as people from various socioeconomic backgrounds, experience ASD. However, compared to females, boys have a much higher risk of developing ASD.

What are a few typical ASD symptoms?
Children with ASD may seem different even as babies, particularly when compared to

other kids their same age. They could fixate on a few things excessively, seldom establish eye contact, and refrain from chattering to their parents as they normally would. In other instances, kids could grow normally up until their second or third birthday, but after that, they might start to retreat and lose interest in social interaction.

The degree to which a person's everyday functioning is impacted by repetitive patterns of behavior, insistence on sameness in activities and settings, and social communication issues may determine how severe an ASD diagnosis is.

Social dysfunction and communication issues

The difficulty of social relationships is common among those with ASD. Common communication and interaction's give-and-take dynamic may be especially difficult. Children with ASD may not acknowledge their names, avoid making eye contact with others, and only engage with others to further their interests. Children with ASD may prefer to be alone since they often don't know how to play or interact with other kids. It may be challenging for someone with ASD to relate to others' emotions or discuss their own.

People with ASD may speak in a variety of ways, from hardly speaking at all to speaking fluently but in socially unacceptable ways. Some ASD kids may repeat words and phrases, provide illogical responses to inquiries, and have delayed speech and language development. Additionally, individuals with ASD may struggle to use and comprehend non-verbal signs such as gestures, body language, and tone of voice. Young toddlers with ASD, for instance, could not comprehend what it means to wave goodbye. People with ASD may also have a flat, robotic, or sing-song voice and talk about a small number of their preferred subjects without much respect for the listener's interests.

Recurrent and distinctive behaviors

Many kids with ASD exhibit strange or repetitive activities, such as flapping their arms, swaying from side to side, or spinning. They could start to focus on certain details of things, like the wheels on a toy truck. Children may develop an obsessional interest in a specific subject, such as trains or aircraft, for example. Changes to everyday routines, such as an unexpected halt on the way home from school, may be quite difficult for many persons with ASD who appear to thrive on predictability. Some kids could even lose their temper or have emotional outbursts, particularly if they are in an unfamiliar or too stimulating setting.

What conditions are connected to ASD?

Fragile X syndrome, which results in intellectual disability, and tuberous sclerosis, which causes benign tumors to grow in the brain and other vital organs, are two known genetic disorders that are linked to an increased risk for autism. Each of these disorders is caused by a mutation in a single, distinct gene. In recent years, scientists have found other genetic alterations in autistic youngsters, some of which have not yet been termed diseases. Even though each of these illnesses is uncommon, together they may be responsible for 20% or more of all instances of autism.

The likelihood of developing seizures is also greater than usual in those with ASD. Before the age of three, children who have language regression seem to be at increased risk of epilepsy or brain activity that resembles seizures. By the time they are adults, 20 to 30 percent of children with ASD have seizures. Additionally, seizure disorders are most likely to occur in persons with ASD and intellectual impairment.

How is ASD identified?

Depending on how severe the illness is, ASD symptoms may differ substantially from person to person. For young children with moderate ASD or other less severe disabilities, symptoms may potentially go unnoticed.

The Diagnostic and Statistical Manual of Mental Illnesses-V, a manual developed by the American Psychiatric Association for the diagnosis of mental disorders, states that autism spectrum disorder is diagnosed by clinicians based on symptoms, signs, and tests. Children should have routine screenings for developmental delays, and in particular, for autism, during their 18- and 24-month well-child visits.

Very early warning signs that need professional assessment include:

by age 1, there must be no chattering or pointing, no single words by 16 months, and no two-word sentences by 2 years.

no reaction to name; loss of previously learned language or social abilities; lack of eye contact

excessive toy or item stacking

no grin or attempt at social interaction

Future signs include:

Lack of creative and social play or its impairment repetitive or unusual language usage excessively strong or concentrated attention concerned with particular items or themes rigid adherence to prescribed routines or rituals poor ability to establish or maintain a conversation with others

A more thorough assessment is often recommended if screening tools suggest the potential of ASD. A multidisciplinary team composed of a psychologist, neurologist, psychiatrist, speech therapist, and other specialists who diagnose and treat ASD in children is necessary for a thorough examination. A comprehensive neurological evaluation as well as in-depth cognitive and linguistic tests will be performed by the team members. Children with delayed speech development should also have their hearing evaluated since hearing issues might result in behaviors that could be misconstrued for ASD.

What brings on ASD?

ASD is thought to be influenced by both genetics and the environment, according to scientists. The fact that autism rates have been rising in recent decades without a clear explanation for why is causing tremendous worry. Numerous genes linked to the illness have been discovered by researchers. Those with ASD exhibit different patterns of brain growth, according to imaging studies. According to studies, changes in normal brain growth very early in development may be the cause of ASD. These disruptions might be the consequence of genetic flaws that affect the genes that direct brain development and govern intercellular communication. Children who were born too soon are more likely to have autism. Even though no particular environmental causes have yet been found, environmental variables may potentially affect how genes operate and evolve. It has long been shown that parenting styles do not cause autism spectrum disorder (ASD). Numerous studies have shown that immunization against infectious illnesses in children does not raise the population's risk of autism.

What function do genes serve?

Twin and family studies provide compelling evidence that certain individuals are predisposed to autism genetically. According to studies of identical twins, the likelihood that the second twin would have the same problem as the first twin ranges from 36 to 95 percent. Numerous research is being conducted to identify the precise genetic variables connected to the development of ASD. The likelihood of having a second kid with ASD rises in homes where there is already one affected child. Numerous genes discovered to be linked to autism have a role in how the chemical connections between brain neurons operate (synapses). Finding hints about the genes that promote vulnerability is a goal of research. Sometimes the parents or other family members of an ASD kid exhibit modest communication disorders in social situations or engage in repetitive actions. Evidence also points to a higher than usual prevalence of emotional illnesses in the relatives of persons with ASD, including bipolar disorder and schizophrenia.

De novo, or spontaneous, gene mutations have also been demonstrated to affect the likelihood of developing autism spectrum disorder, in addition to inherited genetic abnormalities that are found in virtually all of a person's cells. De novo mutations, which may happen spontaneously in a parent's sperm or egg cell or after conception, are alterations in DNA sequences, the human body's genetic material. Then, when the fertilized egg divides, the mutation takes place in each cell. These mutations might damage a single gene or they can cause what are known as copy number variations, which include the deletion or duplication of sections of DNA that contain many genes. Recent research has shown that individuals with ASD tend to have more copy number de novo gene mutations than individuals without the disorder, which suggests that for some individuals, the risk of developing ASD may not be caused by mutations in specific genes but rather by spontaneous coding mutations across several genes. De novo mutations may be used to explain genetic illnesses in which the afflicted kid has the mutation in every cell but none of the parents do, and in which the condition does not run in the family. Children born to older parents are likewise more likely to have autism. To ascertain the possible impact of environmental variables on spontaneous mutations and how it affects the risk of ASD, there is still more study to be done.

Do autistic symptoms evolve?
Many children's symptoms go better as they become older and get behavioral therapy. Some adolescents with ASD may develop depression or behavioral issues at this time, and their therapy may need to be modified as they get older. However, depending on the degree of the disease, persons with ASD may be able to work effectively, live independently, or live in a supportive setting. People with ASD often continue to require services and support as they age.

How does autism therapy work?
There is currently no treatment for ASD. Specific symptoms may be significantly improved with the use of therapies and behavioral interventions, which are intended to treat particular symptoms. Medication may be used to address certain

symptoms. The best treatment strategy integrates treatments and therapies to address each patient's unique requirements. The majority of medical experts agree that the sooner the intervention, the better.

Early behavioral and educational therapies have shown to be highly effective for many children with ASD. Applied behavioral analysis, which promotes good behaviors and discourages bad ones, is one of the highly organized, rigorous skill-oriented training sessions used by therapists in these treatments to assist children in developing social and linguistic abilities. Additionally, family therapy for the parents and siblings of ASD patients typically helps families deal with the unique difficulties of raising an ASD kid.

Chapter 2

Signs of ASD

young children with autism
Early warning signs of autism in children include:

ignoring their name and avoiding making eye contact
refusing to grin when you do
repetitive bodily gestures, such as flapping their hands, flicking their fingers, or swaying their bodies, being less talkative than other kids, repeating the same phrases, and becoming extremely agitated if they dislike a certain flavor, smell, or sound
older children with autism
Autism symptoms in older kids include:

Not being able to express their feelings easily, liking a strict schedule and becoming upset if it changes, having a strong interest in a particular topic or activity, finding it difficult to make friends or preferring to be alone, and taking things literally, such as not understanding expressions like "break a leg."

Autism in both boys and girls

Autism may sometimes manifest differently in males and girls.

For instance, autistic females may be more reserved, conceal their emotions, and seem to handle social settings better.

Thus, it may be more difficult to detect autism in females.

Chapter 3

Parenting kids with ASD

There are basic, commonplace things that may make a difference in addition to the medical treatment and therapies you may arrange for your child or relative.

Concentrate on the good. Children with autism spectrum disorder often react effectively to positive reinforcement, just like everyone else. It follows that when you compliment them for the positive actions they exhibit, it will make both of you feel good.

So that they understand precisely what you appreciated about their actions, be explicit. Seek opportunities to thank them, whether it be with more playtime or a simple gift like a sticker.

Prize your kid for who they are, just as you would with anybody, autistic or not. It's important to accept your kid as they are as a parent.

Be consistent and punctual. People with autism like routines. Make sure they get direction and engagement regularly so they can put what they learn in treatment into practice.

They may use their knowledge in many contexts and acquire new skills and behaviors more quickly as a result. Try to agree on a set of strategies and ways of contact with their therapists and instructors so you can use what they are teaching at home.

Put the play on the agenda. Your youngster may open up and develop a relationship with you if you can find things that are just plain enjoyable rather than more educational or therapeutic.

Allow some time. As you search for the best course of action for your kid, you'll probably test out a wide range of methods, therapies, and strategies. If they don't react well to a certain approach, have a good attitude and try not to become disheartened.

Involve your youngster in daily activities. It could seem simpler to keep your kid out of particular places if they exhibit unexpected behavior. However, by accompanying them on routine tasks like grocery shopping or post office runs, you may be able to assist them to acclimate to their surroundings.

Get assistance. Support from other families, professionals, and friends may be very beneficial, whether it is provided online or in person. Gather a group of loved ones and friends who are familiar with your child's condition. Your kid will need assistance in sustaining his or her friendships since maintaining them may be challenging. Support groups may be a useful method to meet other parents facing comparable difficulties, exchange information, and get assistance. Counseling for couples, families, or individuals may also be beneficial. Ask for assistance and consider what may make your life a bit simpler.

Investigate respite care. This is when your kid is cared after by another person for a while, either within your house, outdoors, or both, so that you may take a little break. You'll need it, particularly if your kid has severe demands as a result of ASD. This may provide you the opportunity to engage in activities that improve your health and that you love, enabling you to return home ready to assist.

These techniques may be used to choose or create your respite support team:

Ask your friends, relatives, and other parents you know for any possible support links.

For suggestions or references, speak with your child's physicians, therapists, and educators. For example, a teacher's assistant you truly like could adore watching children in their spare time.

Additionally, you may advertise for child care assistance in local religious groups, newspapers, online, and at schools and institutions close to you. Make sure you thoroughly review all references.

Become a member of a support group for parents of autistic kids. Learn from what has worked for others. A local autism support center may help you identify self-help groups; alternatively, you can search online.

Ensure your well-being. You must maintain peak physical and mental health as a caregiver to be able to handle the obstacles that arise daily. This calls for taking your time and finding methods to look after yourself so that you have enough of yourself (physically, psychologically, and emotionally) to share.

Be less stressed. ASD parents often experience higher levels of stress than parents of children with other disorders. Caretakers may experience relationship breakdowns and even psychiatric problems if the problem is not addressed. Your health might also be impacted by stress. Keep your affairs to keep from being overburdened. This entails setting aside time each day for oneself. Among the crucial and even enjoyable methods to achieve it are:

Determine the true origins of your stress. If you're feeling overwhelmed, divide your main problems into smaller, more manageable portions. You'll have a strategy and feel better.

Other options include meditation. Be mindful of your inner dialogue as much as your ideas. You'll be able to eliminate pointless concerns.

Exercise. You are not required to visit the gym. Swim, exercise in the yard, dance in the kitchen, or just go for a walk. These are quick and efficient methods to work out.

Take an exercise class if you want some adult companionship. It's a fantastic way to make new friends and get your energy back.

There is no substitute for a restful night's sleep when it comes to rejuvenating your body and mind. Use meditation or relaxation techniques to aid in your relaxation if necessary. That might aid in getting your body ready for sleep.

Be inventive with your cuisine. You probably put a lot of effort into making sure your kid eats well-balanced meals. How are you doing? Consider experimenting with new fruits, vegetables, and cuisines to spice up your unique food. To keep things fresh, look for new recipes. and adhere to a daily eating routine. You can keep your system on track and your energy levels up.

Get your life in order. This is the secret to overcoming obstacles in life while maintaining a good standard of living. You and your family will all gain. Schedule some time each week for mingling and having fun. To bring balance to your hectic days, try these suggestions:

Locate your pals. You do have a kid with special needs. But you are also a person. Being aware of your individuality helps you be a better parent. Spend some time laughing and reuniting with your buddies. You'll be happy that you did.

Rekindle previous interests. Find your knitting needles, clean the piano, or take the golf clubs out of the bag. Try out some new hobbies that interest you.

Count to five each day. Spending a few additional minutes in the morning may help you focus and set the tone for the rest of the day. Consider taking a long, warm shower, gathering your thoughts, or writing down some ideas in a diary.

Do it quickly. Can your spouse or other family members temporarily take up the role of parent? You may get some much-needed alone time by taking a simple stroll around the block or a short trip to the shop.

Chapter 4

How to help your child with day to day life

Use your kid's name when you talk to them so they know who you are

language should be concise and straightforward.

Converse plainly and slowly

Simple hand motions or visuals might help to illustrate what you're saying.

Give your youngster more time to comprehend what you have spoken.

Ask the autism evaluation team whether a speech and language therapist can assist (SLT)

consider using Makaton, PECS, or Signalong to help kids communicate read more communication advice for parents from the National Autistic Society.

Do not attempt to refrain from asking your youngster many questions.

When there is noise, try not to talk.

Don't say words like "pull your socks up" or "break a leg" since they might signify various things to different people.

How to handle anxiety

Both children and adults with autism often struggle with anxiety. It's often brought on by their inability to understand what is happening around them.

Try to determine the cause of your child's anxiety.

It might be as a result of:

A regular change might help your kid be ready for any change, like a change in class at school.

Take your youngster to a more serene location, such as another room, if they are in a busy or colorful area.

Ask your kid's mental health team or the autism assessment team for a recommendation to a counselor or therapist who has expertise with autism if your child exhibits signs of anxiety often. aiding in modifying your child's behavior

Some autistic kids exhibit the following behaviors:

A kind of repeated behavior is called stimming (such as flapping their hands or flicking their fingers)

Meltdowns are absolute losses of control brought on by an extreme overload

Read our suggestions on how to deal with your child's behavior if they exhibit certain behaviors.

eating challenges
A lot of kids are "fussy eaters."

Children with autism may:

eat insufficiently or excessively due to issues with choking or coughing when eating or because they are constipated, which causes them to feel full even though they are not
Keeping a food journal that details what, when, and where your child eats may be beneficial. This might aid in identifying any common problems your kid may have.

Talk to your child's doctor or the autism assessment team if they are experiencing any issues with eating.

The National Autistic Society gives more information on how to assist with eating issues.

difficulty sleeping

Many autistic kids have trouble falling asleep and often wake up throughout the night.

This might be due to:

fear of bright lights from cellphones or tablets
issues with the melatonin sleep hormone
Your kid will benefit if you:

maintaining a sleep journal of your child's sleep patterns will help you identify any trends.
maintaining a consistent sleep schedule, ensuring sure their bedroom is quiet and dark, and allowing them to use earplugs if necessary
If none of these suggestions work, speak with your doctor, who could recommend melatonin as a sleep aid for your kid.

maintaining health

Your youngster must have routine examinations from the:

addressing your child's dental, optical, and medical concerns
A yearly health checkup is required for children over 14 who also have a learning handicap.

Do not be hesitant to ask the staff what they can do to make it simpler for you to see the doctor.

Visit the National Autistic Society for additional information on healthy living.

relationships and interaction
Some autistic kids have trouble making friends.

Some actions you can do to assist include:

Do consult other parents on forums or in nearby support groups for advice.

Consult the school to see if they can assist.

Find out whether the autism assessment team can assist your kid with communication and socialization.

join regional organizations that support people with autism

read more friendship guidance from Ambitious about Autism.

Do not place an excessive amount of pressure on your youngster since developing social skills takes time.

if your kid prefers to be alone, don't push them into social settings.

Chapter 5

How to help your child's behavior
Commonly seen behaviors in kids with autism
Some autistic kids may act out in ways that are very stressful for you and your family.

Some behaviors may be referred to as "difficult" by healthcare practitioners.

These actions consist of:

A kind of repeated behavior is called stimming.
A total loss of control over behavior is known as a meltdown.
Some autistic youngsters may also exhibit verbal or physical aggression. Their actions could be damaging to them or others.

But keep in mind that every autistic kid is unique, so not every day will be difficult or stressful.

Why do these actions occur
Children with autism often struggle with communicating, which may have an impact on their behavior.

These behaviors may result from a variety of factors, such as:

being very sensitive to stimuli such as loud sounds or bright lighting
being less sensitive to touch or pain, experiencing anxiety, particularly when routines abruptly alter, and not being able to make sense of what is happening around them while they are ill or in pain
You and your kid are not to blame for these actions.

Stimming
"Stimulating behavior" is what the term "stimming" refers to. It's a certain pattern of behavior.

Typical stimming actions include:

head-banging, leaping, whirling, and rocking
flicking rubber bands with hands, fingers, and flicking motions
repeating phrases or noises, or focusing on spinning or moving objects
Typically, stimming is not harmful. Even though it could seem strange to others, there's no reason to stop it if it's not bothering you or your kid.

More information about stimming and repeated behaviors may be found in Ambitious about Autism.

Meltdowns A complete loss of control brought on by being completely overloaded is known as a meltdown.

The most crucial thing to do while your kid is having a meltdown is to attempt to remain calm and keep them safe.

Try to hold your kid to keep them safe if you fear they could damage themselves.

While it may not always be feasible to stop meltdowns, there are certain things you may do that could be beneficial.

These consist of:

allowing your kid to use headphones to listen to soothing music, dimming or eliminating harsh lighting, and
preparing in advance for any normal change, such as taking an alternative route to school
Keep a notebook for a few weeks to see if you can identify any situations that might lead to meltdowns and take preventative action.

www.ingramcontent.com/pod-product-compliance
Lightning Source LLC
LaVergne TN
LVHW052110160826
845678LV00015B/3470